Dr. Del's RAPID FATLOSS Meal Plan

A Science Based Eating Strategy for Building Your Leanest Body Ever

Features:
- A Complete Eight-Week Fat Loss Meal Plan
- Six Different Meal Plans Based on Daily Caloric Intake
- Detailed Weekly Shopping Lists
- Separate Muscle Building and Fat Loss Meal Plans

Del Millers, PhD

Author of:
- *Dr. Del's Rapid Fatloss Manual*
- *Dr. Del's Rapid Fatloss Meal Plan*
- *Dr. Del's Rapid Fatloss Cookbook*
- *Dr. Del's Rapid Fatloss Detox-Cleanse Program*
- *Simply DELicious: 10-Minute Meals Cookbook*
- *Del's 10-Minute Workout*
- *Dancing with God*

Dr. Del's Rapid Fatloss Meal Plan
A Science Based Eating Strategy for Building Your Leanest Body Ever

Del Millers, PhD

Published by

Spiritwind Publications
10736 Jefferson Blvd., # 693
Culver City, CA 90230 U.S.A.
888-800-9463

Publisher's Cataloging-in-Publication Data

Millers, Del.
Dr. Del's rapid fatloss meal plan : a science-based eating strategy for building your leanest body ever / Del Millers.
p. cm.
ISBN: 978-0-9666704-9-3
1. Weight loss. 2. Grocery shopping. 3. Nutrition—Popular works. I. Title.
RM222.2 .M5248 2012
613.2`5—dc22
2012904102

Design by Linda Björk
Photographs Michael Burr

Printed in the United States of America

Dedicated to all the members
and future members of the
Living Lean club.

"Before anything else,
preparation is the key to success."
~ *Alexander Graham Bell*

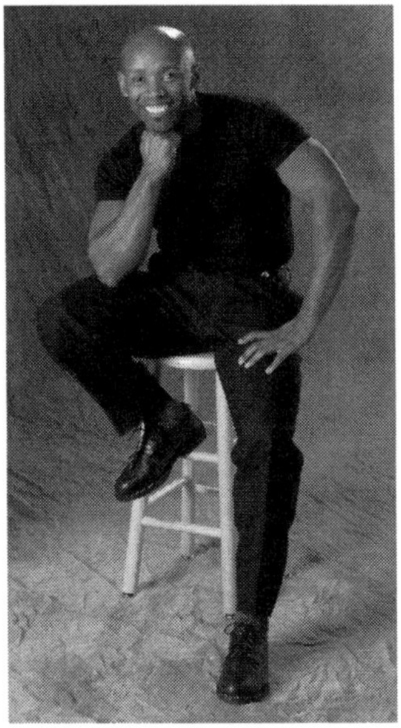

"How you look is a consequence of how you live."
~ Del Millers

Table Of Contents

6 A Note From Dr. Del

9 Profile of Success

11 The Rapid Fatloss Meal Plan

- *11 The Eight Principles Of Success*
- *15 You Need Smart Supplementation*

18 How Many Calories Should You Eat?

- *18 BMR (Basal Metabolic Rate)*
- *20 Your Total Daily Calories*
- *22 How Many Calories Should You Eat?*
- *23 How Not To Count Calories And Still Know How Much To Eat*

24 Meal Frequency: How Many Meals Should You Eat Daily?

27 Macronutrients: Best Sources Of Protein, Carbohydrates & Fats

- *27 Best Sources Of Lean Protein*
- *28 Best Sources Of Complex Carbohydrates*
- *29 Healthy Fats & Oils*
- *30 Vegetables*
- *31 Fruit*
- *32 Using Herbs/ Spices*
- *33 Meal Replacement & Protein Powder*
- *34 Vegan/Vegetarians*

36 8-Week Fat Loss Meal Plan

- *36 Phase One: 21-Day Detox Cleanse*
- *36 Phase Two: Muscle Building & Fitness (3 Weeks)*
- *47 Phase Three: Fat Loss (2 Weeks)*

54 The Key To Your Success: Strive For Consistency, Not Perfection!

56 About The Author

Dr. Del's Personal Mission Statement:

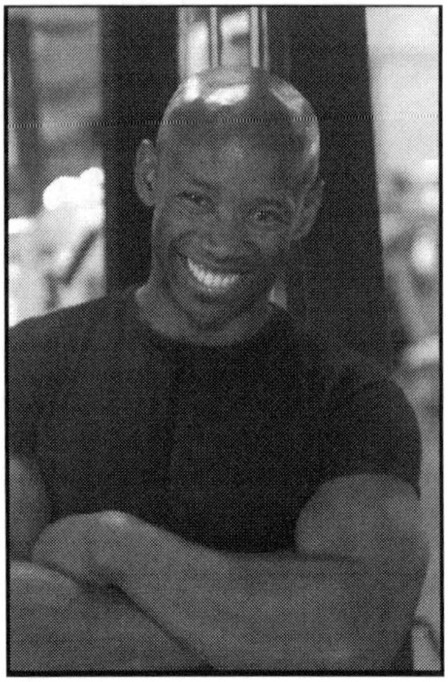

To Inspire, Support and Encourage Personal Growth & Transformation through Health Conscious Living.

A Note From Dr. Del

Many years ago when I first started out as a personal trainer I didn't know very much about nutrition. My clients didn't know very much about nutrition either. So it was the classic case of the blind leading the blind.

However, to my advantage I had great teachers around me. Two of my first teachers were registered dietitians Dr. Marilyn Joyce, RD and Deborah Rude, RD. They were both very instrumental in crafting the early nutrition programs that I shared with my clients.

I soon realized, however, that I had to upgrade my knowledge of nutrition if I was going to successfully help my clients achieve their fitness and weight loss goals. A few years later, I completed my doctoral studies in nutritional sciences.

Health, fitness & body transformation

One of the most important lessons that you need to learn from this book is that what you eat is the key to unlocking the door to your success.

Whether you're trying to lose weight, build muscle, get lean or perform better, you will never achieve significant results without first figuring out what kind of meal plan is best for your specific goals.

Don't make the mistake that most people make in thinking that you can change your body just by eating healthy foods.

There are big differences between health, fitness and body transformation.

For one thing, you can be healthy and not fit. You can also be fit and overweight. If you want to be healthy, focus on what you need to eat to get healthy. If you want to be fit, focus on how you need to eat to achieve your fitness goals.

However, if you want to change your body, you need a body changing meal plan. The same goes for athletic training.

I like to remind my clients that change is temporary, only transformation lasts forever.

What's the difference, you ask? Well, your weight changes everyday based on a lot of variables. Is this a great way to gauge your results? Not in my book.

However, transforming your body requires that you develop new habits and maintain those new healthier habits over time. This is lasting because you can't transform your body without also transforming your life.

That's why I usually tell people at my seminars that "it's not about your body; it's about your life."

To transform your body, you have to put your body and your life through a complete remodeling program.

First, you have to get the body healthy. This means getting the body's various systems (digestion, assimilation, absorption, elimination, hormonal, etc.) functioning optimally. This is the focus of my ***21-Day Detox-Cleanse Program***.

Next you have to build new lean muscle tissue and get much fitter than you currently are. Why? Because this is the most effective way of burning fat, increasing your metabolism and maintaining the results you achieve over time.

So if your goal is to look lean, why are you spending hours on the treadmill? Go lift some weights to build lean muscle then do a short high intensity interval cardio session (HIIT).

The research is conclusive that this is the best way to train for maximum fat burning. I wrote about this in detail in ***Dr. Del's Rapid Fatloss Manual***.

The tricky thing, however, is that you can't train or eat the same way all the time. Your body needs to be shocked and surprised. You have to change how you train and eat regularly for best results.

This is why I developed my Three-Phase training and eating plan.

During Phase One (21-Day Detox-Cleanse Program) the focus is on getting the body healthy.

The focus of Phase Two (Muscle Building & Fitness) is building lean muscle and improving your overall fitness level. Fit, lean people burn more fat doing the exact same activity than their unfit and less lean counterparts.

So why waste time focusing on weight loss? Focus instead on changing your body composition.

In Phase Three, I will show you how to eat to maximize short-term fat loss. This is what I did in the weeks leading up to a bodybuilding contest, though not as restrictive.

As I've said so many times before, change is not only important, it is necessary if you really want to maximize your results.

The meal plan that I have outlined in this book is based on both research and experience. Those who follow it, get results.

This is the same eating strategy I use several times a year to look my best before attending several major speaking and coaching events. I always train to look my best before attending an event, especially those with pool parties.

Hopefully, the next time I see you at one of these events, you'll be looking your best too.

Eat well and prosper.

Del Millers

Profile of Success

NAOMI PESSIN
Culver City, California

Fourteen years ago I met Del Millers, little did I know that we both would make a dramatic change in my life. I lost 63 pounds and kept it off. I'm stronger in mind and body. I'm also a happier person and feel great about myself.

Thanks Del, for giving me the extra push to change.

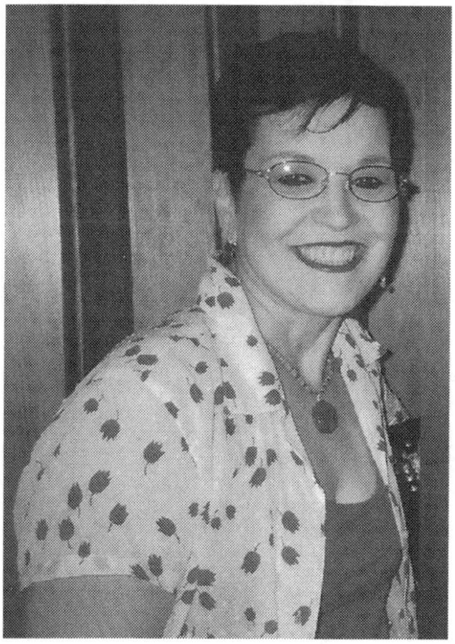

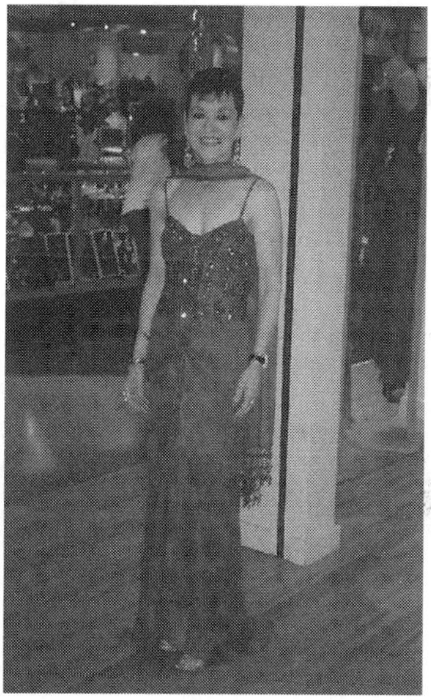

Note
After 14 years, Naomi is still training with me twice per week. How's that for a commitment to a fit lifestyle?

JOANNE BAKER
Marina Del Rey, California

I first met Dr. Del over ten years ago and together we have completely transformed my life. I've lost almost 80 pounds and kept it off.

After a lifetime of being overweight and sedentary, a normal week for me now includes at least two days of weight training with Del, running 3 miles a couple of mornings, at least one 35 mile bike ride on the weekend, if not two, and a five mile hike on Friday nights.

Del has taught me a great deal about weight training, cardio, nutrition, and myself. If faced with a more difficult athletic challenge – say a black diamond ski trail I've never tried before, I take a deep breath, steady my nerves and go for it! I know I have the strength, balance and endurance to handle almost anything. My muscles may groan, but I have Del's smiling face, silently encouraging me to be the best I can be.

Thanks Dr. Del!

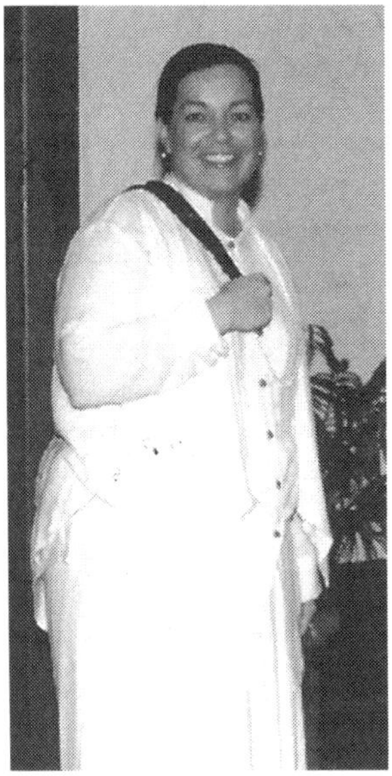

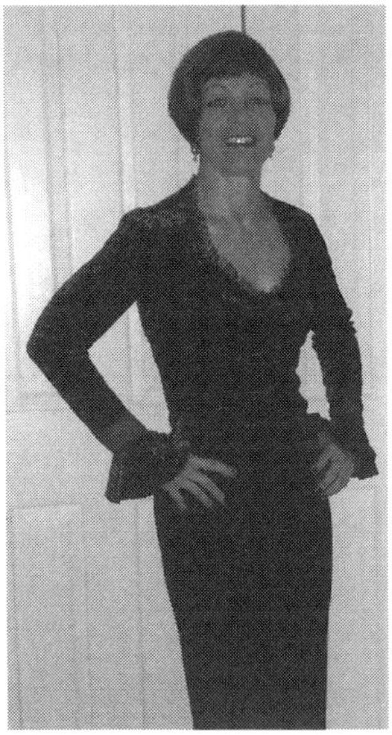

Note
After 11 years, Joanne is also still training with me twice per week. She has become one of the most active people I know. How's that for a life transformation?

The Rapid Fatloss Meal Plan

As I've said before, 80% of changing your body will largely depend on what you eat. Over the past twenty years that I've been working with clients, I've made a few observations I'd like to share with you. The people who are successful in changing their bodies all adhere to a few important fundamentals that I call The Eight Principles of Success.

▼ The Eight Principles of Success

❶ *Follow a Meal Plan*

The most frustrating thing about working with clients is their inability to follow a meal plan. Everyone usually starts off very enthusiastic about their new journey. However, only a few have the ability to weather the storms of life and stay the course.

From my experience, there are three types of clients:

a. The Well-Intentioned

There are those who tell themselves that they want to change their bodies, but they're not READY to do what it takes. And they're not ready for a variety of reasons (work, family, emotional, etc.).

They'll keep trying, as they should, but like I said, they're not READY to do what it takes. The problem with this group is that they don't have a deep emotional reason for wanting to change their bodies. So until they find that BIG WHY or reason, they'll keep trying, but unfortunately they will end up right where they began.

b. The UnCoachable

These are folks who can't stick with anything long enough to determine whether or not they're even moving in the right direction. They'll agree to follow a certain plan, but next week they'll be doing it their way.

Unfortunately, these people will never arrive at their destination because they don't trust that any particular plan can get them there. So they end up chasing their own tails.

c. *The UnStoppable*

These are the folks who get results.

They get results because they're READY to do WHATEVER it takes to get results. They don't make excuses. These people willingly surrender themselves to the process.

Their motto is: "just tell me what to do." They have the ability to follow a plan consistently over time. They possess a kind of single-mindedness of purpose, meaning that they know what they want and nothing can stop them. So even when they are thrown off course, they get up and get right back to it.

To be successful, you have to be able to follow your plan no matter what's going on in your personal or professional life.

❷ *Take Control of Your Habits*

Someone once said "habits are like a comfortable bed, easy to get into but hard to get out of." And isn't that the truth. However, if your goal is to be lean, you have to develop "lean" habits.

You have to completely change your relationship with food. That doesn't mean giving up eating the things you love, that's deprivation, and it doesn't work. But you have to realize the difference between a "treat" and a "habit."

If you're eating pizza two or three times per week, that's not a treat, it's a pizza eating habit. Having a "cheat" meal once per week is a treat. Or saving up your cheat meals and going to a really nice restaurant once a month is a treat.

Now that sounds like a great treat to me, which is what I do. Once a month, I go out to sushi or to a really nice restaurant.

❸ *Make It Happen; Don't Make Excuses*

You're not going to change your body by making excuses. Either you do your cardio or you don't. You either follow your meal plan or you don't. But if you don't, stop expecting to see results.

❹ *Set Attainable Short Term Goals*

It's a lot easier to wrap your head around losing ten pounds than it is to focus on losing fifty. Get in the habit of working on small goals at a time. If you're trying to lose weight, focus on ten pounds at a time.

Lose the first ten then set another goal to lose the next ten. If you're just trying to get leaner, follow the process of building as much muscle as you can in a 4-week period using my Phase Two guidelines, then spend the next two weeks on my Phase Three fat loss plan.

Keep going back and forth between the two phases until you reach your goal.

❺ *Reward Yourself*

Enjoy the journey. Put yourself in training for a period of time then reward yourself. Go to a special restaurant, a spa, buy a new outfit, whatever excites you. Don't just beat yourself up, add rewards as part of the process.

❻ *Develop a Lifestyle Around Your Goals*

If you're always trying to squeeze fitness into your busy, chaotic lifestyle, chances are you will always be struggling. Think about it, when your shoes fit comfortably you don't really think about your feet do you?

Likewise, those who tend to successfully get the results they're looking for don't think much about fitness and healthy eating, they just do it. They've developed a lifestyle around being lean.

That means if they have to get up at 5 am in the morning to workout, they will. They consciously change their lives around so that they may do what they need to do to maintain a lean, fit and healthy lifestyle.

❼ *Stay off the Cardio Machines*

Here's an eye opener for you. Why would you waste your time walking for an hour when you can get a better more effective fat burning workout in half the time? Just twenty to thirty minutes of high intensity interval training will super-charge your fat burning system more efficiently than walking for an hour.

The research is conclusive, we've proven this to be a fact, so stop wasting your time. Train hard and then go enjoy the rest of your life.

❽ *Take Time Off*

Yes, that's right. It's important to take time off from training. This not only keeps you fresh, it also prevents burnout. One suggestion is to dedicate yourself to a 12-week training program, then take a week off.

If you have to take a business or personal trip, think about using that as your time off then come back and recommit to your plan. Just don't use this as an excuse to take too much time off or you'll never achieve your goal.

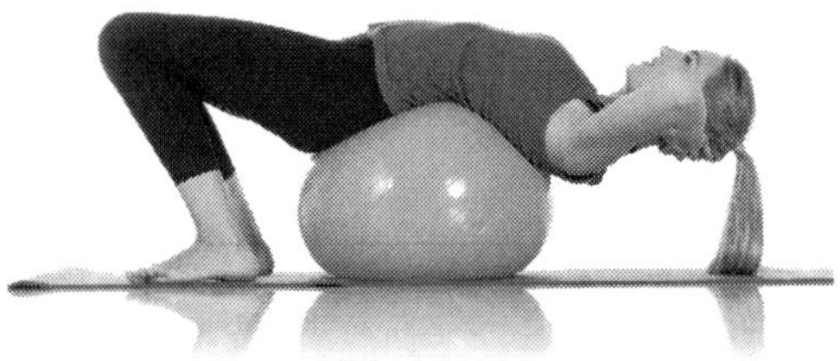

▼ You Need Smart Supplementation

I'm not a big believer in taking a lot of supplements. Having said that, it is almost impossible to build a great looking body without smart supplementation. When you're trying to change your body, your primary objective is to give it everything it needs so that it can do what it needs to do.

During weight loss, you need to minimize the effects of carbohydrate restriction and build up your immune system. You also want to make sure that your body is getting a lot of active enzymes in order to properly metabolize the foods you eat. This can be a problem for a lot of people, especially those with very poor eating habits.

If you're overweight, chances are you haven't exactly been walking the straight and narrow when it comes to making all the right food choices. And the fact that your body is holding on to excess weight should tell you that the body's various systems are not functioning at optimum capacity. By systems I mean digestion, elimination, assimilation, absorption and most importantly, your hormonal system.

The best way to put your body back on track is with a program of whole foods, which is all you will be eating on my meal plan. However, it is not possible to eat all the various varieties of whole foods that you really need to get all the necessary antioxidants, phyto-chemicals (plant chemicals), active enzymes and all the thousands of other great things God gave us in natural foods.

Also keep in mind that the more active you are (and you will be on my program), the more nutrients your body will require to produce fuel for your working muscles, to repair damaged muscles, and to help you recover quickly so that you can continue doing what needs to be done.

Having said all that, here are a few recommendations of things I use with my clients—those who are serious about getting results. I should mention that the clients I work with who are serious about getting results are the ones who follow my recommendations.

And consequently, they get the best results. The others, who like to pay for professional advice then turn around and do their own thing, are the ones who are continually struggling to lose the same ten pounds; go figure.

Note:

You should notice that I'm not in the business of telling you what NOT to do. My primary objective is to share with you what I have found to be effective in creating better health, weight loss and body transformation.

If I don't mention something here, it's because I don't think it's all that important for what you're trying to do. I approach everything from a "less is more" perspective. As such, you really don't need to take half dozen different supplements because they're not going to help you.

Here's what I think may help you:

A Fruit and Vegetable Capsule

A fruit and vegetable juice powder in capsule or chewable form is a great way to flood your body with all those important phyto-chemicals, anti-oxidants and active enzymes that your body so desperately needs to keep all the above mentioned systems functioning optimally.

A recent study published in Medicine & Science in Sports & Exercise Journal, reported that the group that used a fruit and vegetable capsule JuicePlus® had a significant reduction in the breakdown of protein due to the stress caused by exercise.

This is very significant because as I mentioned above, when you're trying to lose weight you want to minimize the loss of lean muscle tissue. By reducing the breakdown of protein you are in essence minimizing the breakdown of lean tissue, which is made up of protein. As a result, not only will you perform better, but you will also build a better body, faster.

Glutamine

Glutamine is another worthwhile supplement that also helps to minimize muscle catabolism (breakdown).

EFA's: You've Got to Eat Fat to Lose Fat

One of the most important things you can do to lose fat is to start eating more healthy fats like olive oil, flax seed oil, primrose oil, avocado and peanut butter. The problem with restricting the good fats is that they also contain Essential Fatty Acids (EFA). And EFA's are responsible for thousands of biological functions throughout the body. Since the body cannot manufacture them, they must be provided by your diet.

EFA's not only help to increase testosterone production, they also aid in the prevention of muscle breakdown, help to increase your HDL level (good cholesterol) and assist in hormone production. For these reasons, I recommend using an essential fatty acid supplement daily. I would recommend using fish oil daily, either the oil or capsules. Flax seeds are also a good source of omega-3 fats, though not as good as fish oil. I discussed this in detail in Dr. Del's Rapid Fatloss Manual.

Unless you're an advance exerciser, anything more than the above would probably be a waste of your money. When you get to a level where you're able to do very intense strength and cardio training, some of the other supplements I reviewed in the Dr. Del's Rapid Fatloss Manual may be useful.

Micronutrients

Micronutrients are nutrients that the body requires in very small quantities to carry out a wide range of physiological functions. These include vitamins, minerals, and thousands of other plant-based chemicals (phytochemicals) that are vital to the fat burning process. For this reason, I recommend using a fruit and vegetable capsule, such as JuicePlus.

How Many Calories Should You Eat?

The amount of calories you will need daily will depend on several factors: your age, weight, height, percent body fat and of course your fitness goals.

▼ BMR (Basal Metabolic Rate)

First things first: let's talk about the minimum amount of calories your body needs daily just to keep you alive. We call this your BMR or Basal Metabolic Rate. That's the amount of calories your body needs for respiration, circulation, to keep your heart beating, your lungs, liver and other vital organs functioning.

Calculating Your BMR

The easiest way to calculate your BMR is simply to add a zero to your weight. For example, a woman who weighs 140 lbs. requires 1400 calories just to keep the body's vital organs functioning...add a zero to 140. A man who weighs 170 lbs. requires at least 1700 calories daily.

NEVER EAT FEWER CALORIES THAN YOUR BMR. IF YOU DO, YOUR BODY WILL START TO FEED ON ITSELF!!! A VERY UGLY EXPERIENCE...

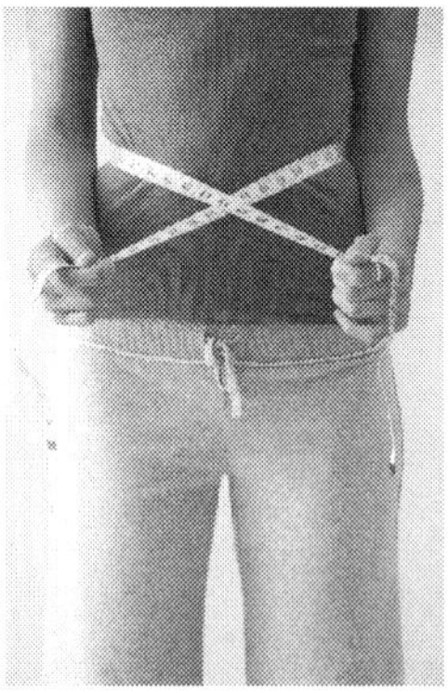

THE HARRIS-BENEDICT EQUATION

(BMR based on total body weight)

MEN: BMR = 66 + (13.7 X wt in kg) + (5 X ht in cm) – (6.8 X age in years)

WOMEN: BMR = 655 + (9.6 X wt. in kg) + (1.8 X ht in cm) – (4.7 X age in years)

Note: 1 inch = 2.54 cm / 1 Kilogram = 2.2 lbs.

EXAMPLE:
You are a female
You are 35 years old
You are 5′5″ tall (65 inches = 165.1 cm)
You weigh 140 lbs.. (63.6 kg)

Your BMR = 655 + (9.6 X 63.6) + (1.8 X 165.1) – (4.7 X 35) = 1405 calories/day

Oh but Dr. Del, I know me. I'll never count calories...

Take heart, this information is primarily for those of you who need to accurately calculate your daily caloric needs. If you're not interested in doing these calculations (or just plain won't, or maybe never got higher than a D+ in math) I'll show you an easier way when we get to your meal plan.

Comparison Of Weight-Loss Diets With Different Compositions Of Fat, Protein, And Carbohydrates

Diets with 20% fat, 15% protein & 65% carbohydrates; 20% fat, 25% protein & 55% carbohydrates; and 40% fat, 25% protein, 35% carbohydrates led to the same amount of weight loss after 2 years.

~ *New England Journal of Medicine*

▼ Your Total Daily Calories:

Now that you know your BMR, you can calculate your total amount of calories your body burns each day. We call this your Total Daily Energy Expenditure (TDEE).

TDEE = BMR x Activity Index

EXAMPLE:
Your BMR is 1405
Your Activity Index is 1.8
Your TDEE = 1405 X 1.8 = 2,529 calories

ACTIVITY INDEX

Average Couch Potato	= BMR X 1.2 Sedentary
Light activity	= BMR X 1.4 Light exercise 1-3 days/week
Moderately active	= BMR X 1.6 Moderate exercise 3-5 days/week
Very active	= BMR X 1.8 Hard exercise 6-7 days/week
Intense activity	= BMR X 2.0 Intense workouts or very physical job
Extended intensity	= BMR X 2.5 Extremely high intensity, high duration sports activity

A Simpler Way Of Calculating Your BMR Is Based On Your Lean Body Mass

KATCH-MCARDLE FORMULA

BMR (Men & Women) = 370 + (21.6 x lean mass in kg)
TDEE = BMR X Activity level

This is a more accurate equation if you are either very muscular or very obese. Remember, TDEE is your maintenance level—the daily amount of calories required to maintain your current weight.

TO LOSE FAT WEIGHT:

Reduce Daily Calories (TDEE) by 15-20% = Calorie deficit

EXAMPLE:
Your weight is 140 lbs.
Your TDEE is 2000 calories.
Your Calorie deficit is 20% of TDEE = 400 calories.
Your Optimal Calorie intake for weight loss = 1600 calories.

TO GAIN LEAN MUSCLE:

Increase Daily Caloric intake (TDEE) by 15-20%

EXAMPLE:
Your weight is 140 lbs.
Your TDEE is 2000.
Your Optimal Caloric intake for weight gain = 2000 + (300-400)
= 2300-2400 calories.

▼ How Many Calories Should You Eat?

1 gm. protein = 4 calories
1 gm. fat = 9 calories
1 gm. carbohydrate = 4 calories
1 ounce = 28 gm.

EXAMPLE:
You're interested in fat loss.
Your weight is 140 lbs.
Your TDEE is 2000 calories.
Your Calorie deficit is 20% of TDEE = 400 calories
Your Optimal Calorie intake for weight loss = 1600 calories = TDEE (Optimal)

Protein	= 30%	= .30 X TDEE (Optimal) = 480 cal. divide by 4 = 120gms/day
Carbohydrates	= 50%	= .50 X TDEE (Optimal) = 800 cal. divide by 4 = 200 gms/day
Fat	= 20%	= .20 X TDEE (Optimal) = 500 cal. divide by 9 = 56 gms/day

Again, keep in mind that the types of carbohydrates I recommend you eat are very low in calories and very dense in nutrition. Therefore, you will be able to eat a lot more food without consuming an excessive amount of calories.

> "Regular eating was associated with lower EI (energy intake), greater postprandial thermogenesis (elevated metabolism after a meal), and lower fasting total and LDL ("bad") cholesterol."
> ~ American Journal of Clinical Nutrition

▼ How Not To Count Calories And Still Know How Much To Eat

Let's face it, who likes to sit around counting calories all day? I sure don't and I never do. Even when I was training for natural bodybuilding competition I never counted calories. I ate small balanced meals every two to three hours, and it worked.

I only included the information on how to calculate how many calories you need daily in this book as a reference for those of you who are so inclined to use it. However, it's really not necessary.

The important thing when it comes to changing your body is eating regular balanced meals. How regular? Well, 4-6 times a day is the best way. Eating 4-6 times a day not only gives you energy, it also speeds up your metabolism.

No joke, this is supported by research. A recent study in the European Journal of Clinical Nutrition confirmed that people who ate six times a day had a faster resting metabolic rate than those who ate just three meals a day.

Now what's a balanced meal?

A balanced meal is the right combination of the macronutrients protein, carbohydrates and fats. For example, a good lunch could be a chicken breast, brown rice and a cup of vegetables. Your healthy fat could either be the olive oil you use to cook or a slice of avocado. Another simple meal could be a handful of nuts and a piece of fruit. It's that simple.

As I said before, I never ask my clients to count calories, I do it all for them. All you have to do is follow one of the sample meal plans. It doesn't have to be exact; you can choose your own source of protein and carbs.

The important thing to keep in mind is the portion size of each serving. That's where most people go wrong. They simply eat too much during each meal.

Meal Frequency:

How Many Meals Should You Eat Daily?

"Participants who ate six times a day had a faster resting metabolic rate than those who ate just three meals a day."
~ *European Journal of Clinical Nutrition*

The vast majority of nutrition experts and fitness professionals around the world, including myself, recommend 4-6 meals per day.

However, this has been a source of controversy over the years, for reasons beyond my comprehension. It should be common sense that eating smaller meals more frequently would stabilize your blood sugar and ultimately lead to your body storing less fat. So what's the debate about?

When I was a kid growing up in Jamaica, we ate breakfast, lunch, a mid-afternoon snack and dinner. Even before I was a fitness professional, I realized that if I didn't have breakfast, lunch, a mid-afternoon snack and dinner, I wouldn't have enough energy to make it through the day.

If I left out my mid-afternoon meal or ate a large lunch instead, I would either lose concentration easily because of hunger or I would fall asleep at my desk because of the insulin spike from eating a large meal.

Remember, the job of insulin is to remove excess glucose from your blood. Therefore, a large meal can quickly lead to low blood sugar, which will leave you feeling tired and lethargic.

So why do we need research to tell us what should be common sense?

When you eat smaller meals every three to four hours, you will have more energy, focus and concentration. You will also be more productive at work. This is also the right approach for fat loss.

Several clinical studies have demonstrated that eating frequently throughout the day is the right approach to maximize fat-burning. Eating regular meals lead to a reduction in total insulin secretion, thereby lowering the probability that your body is storing most of the calories you eat as fat. What's the debate about?

Here's one of those studies, published in the British Journal of Nutrition:

"Eating three meals compared with two meals increased 24 h fat oxidation, but decreased the amount of fat oxidized from the breakfast. The same amount of energy divided over three meals compared with over two meals increased satiety feelings over 24 h. In healthy, normal-weight women, decreasing the inter-meal interval sustains satiety, particularly during the day, and sustains fat oxidation, particularly during the night."

Another study published in the International Journal of Obesity & Related Metabolic Disorders concluded:

"Irregular meal frequency led to a lower postprandial energy expenditure (TEF) compared with the regular meal frequency, while the mean energy intake was not significantly different between the two. The reduced TEF with the irregular meal frequency may lead to weight gain in the long term."

If you forgot already, TEF (thermal effect of food) is the rise in metabolism following a meal.

Another study published in the British Journal of Nutrition reported that:

"During the first 3 weeks (of the study), a diet with a high-protein concentration, fed as frequent small meals, is associated with better preservation of lean tissue than an isoenergetic (same) diet with lower-protein concentration fed as fewer meals."

Preserving lean muscle mass while dieting or going through a fat loss program is crucial because muscle tissue directly affects your metabolism.

Studies have demonstrated that leaner men have a higher metabolism than overweight or obese men (American Journal of Physiology).

So here's the bottom line, there's a reason why most lean people eat 4-6 meals per day. And that's because frequent meals lead to better insulin sensitivity, blood glucose and blood lipid profile. That's just a fancy way of saying that you'll end up storing less fat from what you eat by eating frequently.

However, don't get too fanatical about all this stuff. If you were to miss a meal or two one day, it's not the end of the world. Nobody ever gets fat from skipping a couple meals. However, if you really want to get lean, you should strive for consistency.

"Irregular meal frequency led to a lower postprandial energy expenditure (TEF) compared with the regular meal frequency, while the mean energy intake was not significantly different between the two. The reduced TEF with the irregular meal frequency may lead to weight gain in the long term."

~ International Journal of Obesity & Related Metabolic Disorders

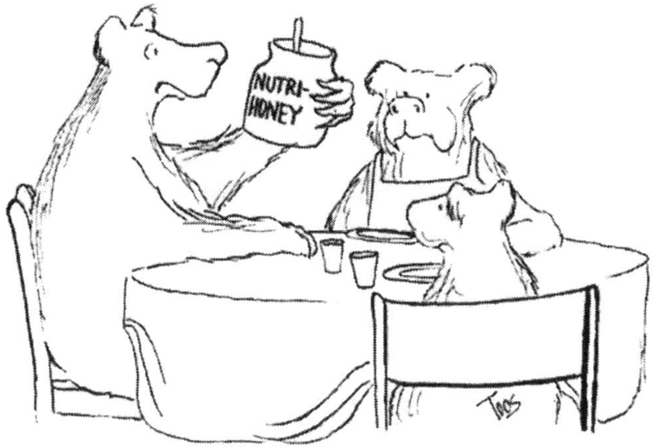

Macronutrients:

Best Sources of Protein, Carbohydrates & Fats

▼ Best Sources of Lean Protein:

What is a serving?

4 oz cooked lean meat
4 oz fish
4 oz chicken breast
4 oz turkey breast
4-oz lean ground turkey
4 oz lean beef (round or sirloin)
2 egg whites, 1 whole egg
1 can tuna (in water)
4 oz wild game—rabbit, venison, pheasant
4 oz veal
4 oz tofu
4 oz tempeh
1/2 cup nonfat cottage cheese
4 oz buffalo
1 can sardine (water or olive oil)
1 cup soybeans (cooked)

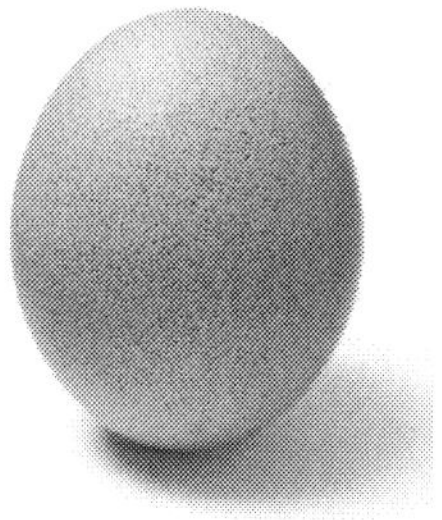

▼ Best Sources of Complex Carbohydrates:

What is a serving?

1/2 cup cooked oatmeal (old fashioned, rolled oats)
1/2 cup cooked brown/wild rice
1/2 cup cooked quinoa
1/2 cup cooked beans, lentils
1/2 cup green peas
1 small baked potato
1 small baked yam
1 cup vegetable soup (home made or store "fresh")
1/2 cup corn
1 cup chopped squash
1 cup plain yogurt
1 cup soy milk
1/2 cup barley, bulgur

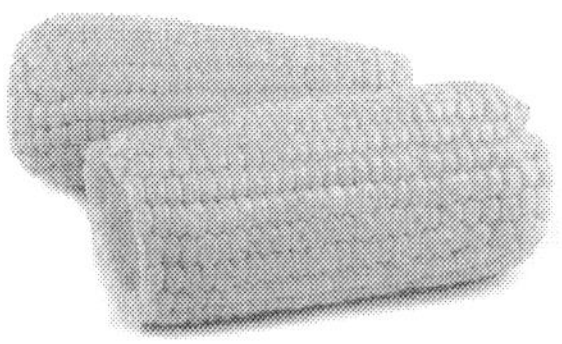

▼ Healthy Fats & Oils

1 oz (1/4 cup) raw unsalted nuts
- almonds
- brazil nuts
- cashew
- hazel nuts
- pine nuts
- walnuts
- pecans
- macadamia
- peanuts

1 tsp. peanut/almond butter
1 tbsp. extra virgin olive/canola oil
1 tbsp. flaxseed oil
1 tbsp. ground flaxseeds
1/4 medium avocado

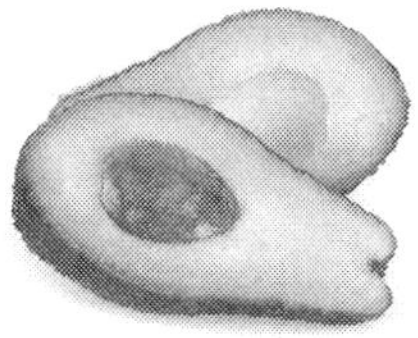

▼ Vegetables

What is a serving?

1/2 cup cooked or 1 cup raw

- asparagus
- beets
- peppers
- broccoli
- spinach
- cauliflower
- mustard greens
- collard greens
- kale
- cabbage
- carrots
- eggplant
- tomato
- bok choy
- brussels sprouts
- green beans
- mushrooms

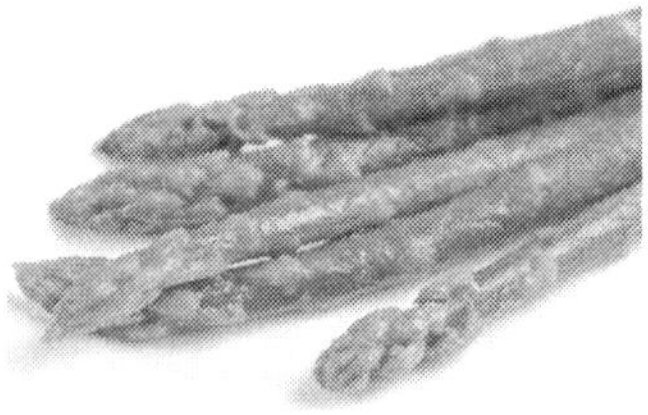

▼ Fruit

What is a serving?

1 medium size fruit
1 cup chopped fruit
- melon
- 1/2 grapefruit
- 2 raw kiwi
- 15 small grapes
- apple
- banana
- berries
- mango
- nectarines
- orange
- papaya
- peach
- pear
- pineapple
- plums
- tangerine

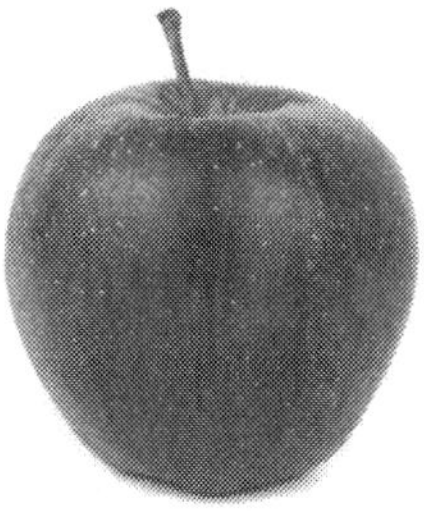

▼ Using Herbs/ Spices:

Bay leaf
Basil
Cinnamon
Cumin
Curry
Garlic
Ginger
Mint
Mustard
Mixed Italian blend
Nutmeg
Onion
Pepper
Thyme
Vanilla extract

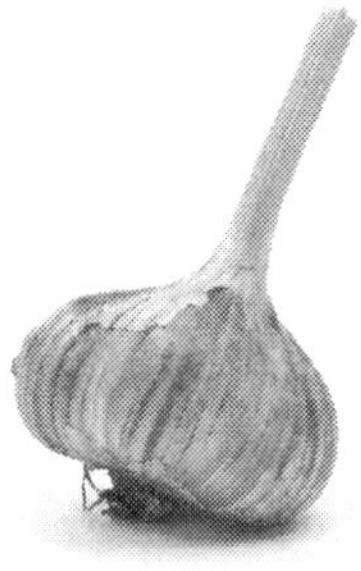

▼ Meal Replacement & Protein Powder:

JuicePlus® Complete Meal Replacement is my first choice (soy based).
Jay Robb Whey/Egg White Protein Powder (with no sugar added).

A Quick Note About Protein Powders:

Choosing the right meal replacement or protein powder can be confusing. If you're interested in bodybuilding, I would recommend going to a nutrition store that caters to bodybuilders because you may want to get one of the many meal replacements that is specifically targeted to bodybuilders.

For everyone else, the JuicePlus® Complete and the Jay Robb should be sufficient. These are the two that I use and recommend to my clients. I use these because they are made with natural whole food ingredients. Additionally, the taste is superior to most others that I have tried.

Whether you choose whey, egg white, casein or vegan protein powder is a matter of personal preference. I have used all types and there is no significant difference between them.

You may also want to consider a meal replacement powder such as the JuicePlus® Complete. Meal replacements are different from protein powders; they contain a balance of carbohydrates, protein and other essential nutrients in a convenient powder form.

Again, I use the JuicePlus® Complete daily because it is made with non-genetically modified soy protein, and it also contains fruit and vegetable juice powder, which is a great source of antioxidants and other essential plant nutrients.

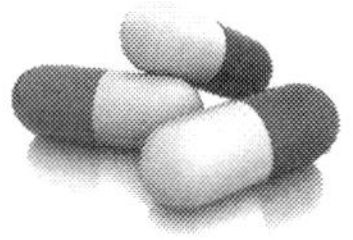

▼ Vegan/Vegetarians

Being a vegan or vegetarian doesn't mean merely cutting out meat and dairy products. If you're a vegan or vegetarian and you're really interested in changing your body, you have to be even more diligent about your meal plan.

Most vegans and vegetarians that I've met all eat too much processed carbohydrates and not enough pure protein. Remember, there's a difference between eating to be healthy and eating to change your body; they're not the same thing.

Eating too many carbohydrates won't help you to get lean because your body has a very limited glycogen storage capacity. However, it has an unlimited fat storage capacity. And excess carbohydrates are easily stored as fat.

The same principles I have outlined in this book apply equally to vegans and vegetarians. However, proper food combination is essential in order to maximize your protein intake and minimize eating a lot of unused carbohydrates.

In Dr. Del's Rapid Fatloss Manual I gave you a simple formula for food combination (My Grandmother Likes Nuts and Seeds) to ensure adequate complete protein intake. Remember, most plant-based sources of protein, with the exception of soy, are not complete proteins because they are missing one or more essential amino acids.

This is not such a big deal. All you have to do is to combine any two complementary foods from the following five categories and you will end up with complete proteins:

1. Milk & dairy (complete protein--egg white is the most perfect protein)
2. Grains
3. Legumes (lentils, beans & peas)
4. Nuts
5. Seeds

Combining foods from any two columns from the table below will give you a complete protein. For example, combining grains and legumes (rice and beans) will give you a complete protein.

Grains	Legumes	Nuts/Seeds
Rice	Beans	Walnuts
Oats	Lentils	Cashews
Barley	Chickpeas	Almonds
Buckwheat		Other nuts
Quinoa		Sesame seeds
Wheat		Pumpkin seeds
Barley		Sunflower seeds
Rye		Other seeds

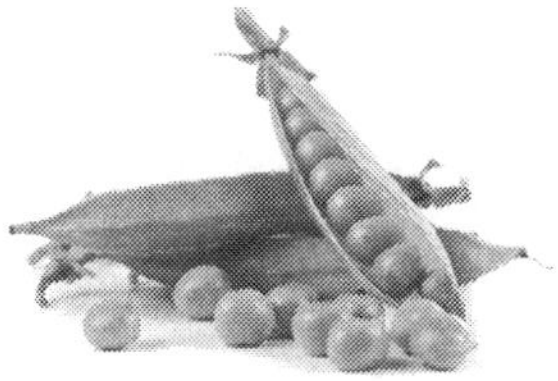

8-Week Fat Loss Meal Plan

▼ PHASE ONE: 21-Day Detox Cleanse

The nutrition plan for this phase will be discussed in Dr. Del's Rapid Fatloss Detox-Cleanse Program.

▼ PHASE TWO: Muscle Building & Fitness (3 Weeks)

Your caloric intake on the meal plan should be 15%-20% higher than during the Fat Loss Phase (Phase 3).

"The composition of diets for body builders should be 55-60% carbohydrate, 25-30% protein and 15-20% of fat, for both the off-season and pre-contest phases. During the off-season the diet should be slightly hyperenergetic (approximately 15% increase in energy intake) and during the pre-contest phase the diet should be hypoenergetic (approximately 15% decrease in energy intake)."

~ Sports Medicine Journal

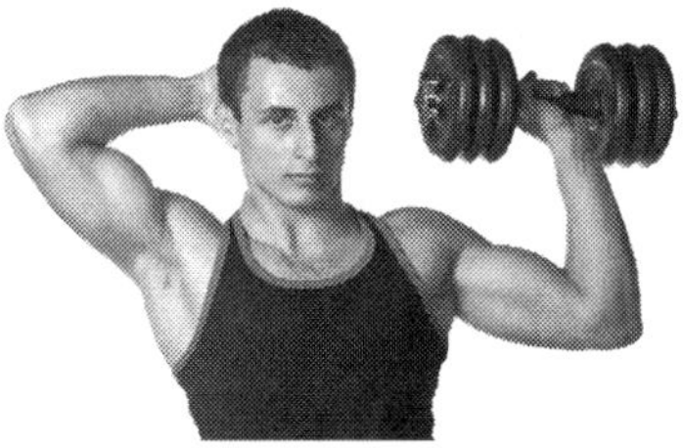

1500 Calories

Meal	Carbohydrate	Protein	Fat	Vegetable	Fruit
Breakfast	1	1	1		1
Lunch	1	1	1	2	
Afternoon		1	1		2
Dinner		1	1	2	

EXAMPLE:
These are just example meals. You can substitute any protein, carbohydrate, fat, fruits and vegetables from the lists above.

Breakfast	Lunch	Mid-Afternoon	Dinner
1/2 cup oatmeal 2 egg whites 1 whole egg 1/2 cup berries 1 tsp peanut butter	4 oz chicken breast 1/2 cup brown rice 1 cup broccoli 1 tsp olive oil	1 banana 1 orange 1/2 cup cottage cheese 12 almonds	4 oz fish 1 cup steamed veggies 1/4 small avocado

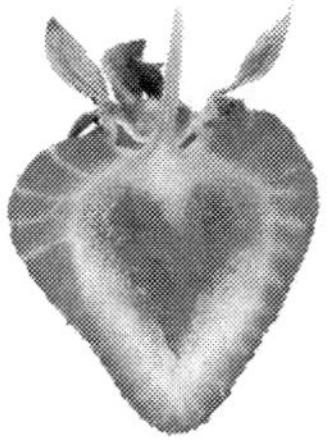

1800 Calories

Meal	Carbohydrate	Protein	Fat	Vegetable	Fruit
Breakfast	1	1	1		1
Lunch	1	2	1	2	
Afternoon	1	1	1		2
Dinner	1	1	1	2	
Anytime			1		1

EXAMPLE:

These are just example meals. You can substitute any protein, carbohydrate, fat, fruits and vegetables from the lists above.

Breakfast	Lunch	Mid-Afternoon	Dinner	Anytime
1/2 cup oatmeal 2 egg whites 1 whole egg 1/2 cup berries 1 tsp peanut butter	8 oz chicken breast 1 medium baked yam 1 cup broccoli 1 tsp olive oil	1 banana 1 orange 1/2 cup cottage cheese 12 almonds	4 oz fish 1 cup brown rice 1 cup steamed veggies 1/4 small avocado	1 tsp peanut/ almond butter 1 apple

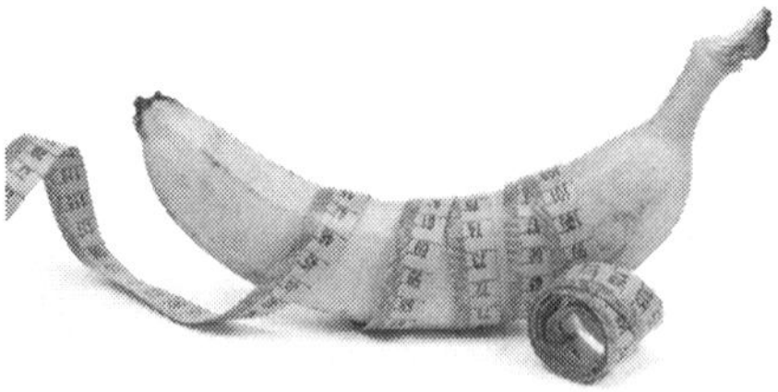

2000 Calories

Meal	Carbohydrate	Protein	Fat	Vegetable	Fruit
Breakfast	1	1	1		1
Lunch	1	2	1	2	
Afternoon	1	1	1		2
Dinner	1	2	1	2	
Anytime		1	1		1

EXAMPLE:
These are just example meals. You can substitute any protein, carbohydrate, fat, fruits and vegetables from the lists above.

Breakfast	Lunch	Mid-Afternoon	Dinner	Anytime
1/2 cup oatmeal 5 egg whites 1 whole egg 1/2 cup berries 1 tsp peanut butter	8 oz chicken breast 1 medium baked yam 1 cup broccoli 1 tsp olive oil	1 banana 1 orange 1 cup cottage cheese 12 almonds	8 oz fish 1 cup brown rice 1 cup steamed veggies 1/4 small avocado	protein smoothie

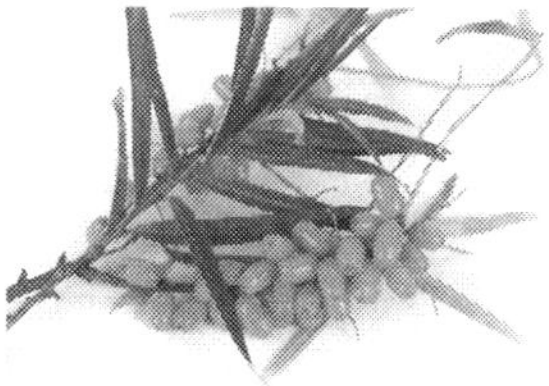

2200 Calories

Meal	Carbohydrate	Protein	Fat	Vegetable	Fruit
Breakfast	1	2	1		1
Lunch	1	2	1	2	
Afternoon	1	2		1	2
Dinner	1	2	1	2	
Anytime	1	2	1		1

EXAMPLE:
These are just example meals. You can substitute any protein, carbohydrate, fat, fruits and vegetables from the lists above.

Breakfast	Lunch	Mid-Afternoon	Dinner	Anytime
1 cup oatmeal 6 egg whites 1 whole egg 1 cup berries 1 tsp peanut butter	8 oz chicken breast 1 medium baked yam 1 cup broccoli 1 tsp olive oil	1 banana 1 orange 1 cup cottage cheese 12 almonds	8 oz fish 1 cup brown rice 1 cup steamed veggies 1/4 small avocado	protein smoothie

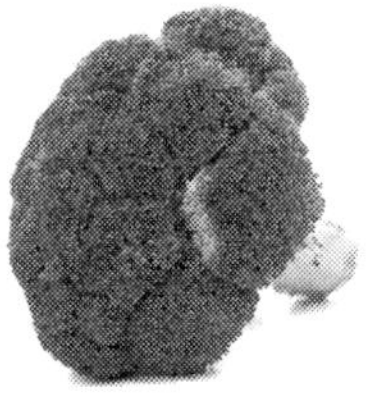

PHASE TWO: Muscle Building & Fitness

Weekly Menu & Shopping List

1500 Calories

(For a 1800 calorie or more meal plans, follow the guidelines above for serving size and number of meals).

Week 1:

A Quick Note: The recipes for all the meals listed below are outlined in ***Dr. Del's Rapid Fatloss Cookbook***. **Also, Day 7 is a FREE DAY.** Go ahead and eat whatever you want.

Meal	Day 1	Day 2	Day 3	Day 4	Day 5	Day 6	Day 7
Breakfast	Toasted Oatmeal w/apple, almonds & banana Juiceplus Fruit Fish Oil	Strawberry-banana tofu smoothie Juiceplus Fruit Fish Oil	Egg white scramble Juiceplus Fruit Fish Oil	Oatmeal & egg white pancakes Juiceplus Fruit Fish Oil	Cottage cheese, yogurt & blueberries Juiceplus Fruit Fish Oil	Yogurt parfait Juiceplus Fruit Fish Oil	Free Day
Lunch	Southwest Turkey or Chicken wrap Juiceplus Vineyard	Shrimp & chicken rice paper wrap w/chili-lime sauce Juiceplus Vineyard	Turkey stir-fry Juiceplus Vineyard	Tuna salad w/apple & avocado Juiceplus Vineyard	Vegetarian chili Juiceplus Vineyard	Salmon cakes w/ sesame gin-ger sauce Juiceplus Vineyard	
Afternoon	Tofu spread	Apple & 16 almonds	Cottage cheese, yogurt & blueberries	Apple & 16 almonds	Hard boiled egg whites & orange	Berrilicious smoothie	
Dinner	Blackened Salmon Juiceplus Veggie Fish oil	Spinach & black-eyed peas Juiceplus Veggie Fish oil	Scallops w/ grapefruit, ginger & miso Juiceplus Veggie Fish oil	Chicken in soy-sherry-sesame reduction Juiceplus Veggie Fish oil	Ginger beef w/broccoli Juiceplus Veggie Fish oil	Apricot chicken w/ almonds Juiceplus Veggie Fish oil	

Week One Shopping List & Other Necessities:

Shopping List	Precooked	Pantry necessities
Chicken breast Salmon fillet Frozen shrimp Eggs Ground turkey Cottage cheese Greek plain non-fat yogurt Scallops Steak Soft silken tofu Firm tofu Low fat cottage cheese Mild salsa Rice paper wrappers (Asian market) Tahini **Fruits & Vegetables:** Apples Oranges Bananas Strawberries Spinach Tomatoes Avocado Red bell pepper Garlic Onions Green onions Large head of lettuce Mushrooms Cilantro Ginger Grapefruit Broccoli	Brown rice Chicken breast Turkey breast	Black-eyed peas Canned tuna Canned salmon Canned black beans Canned kidney beans Canned white beans Canned pinto beans Old fashioned oats Soymilk (unsweetened) Raisins Protein Powder (JuicePlus Complete) Ground flax meal Peanut/almond butter Sliced almonds Canned diced tomatoes Tomato paste Whole wheat flour Natural muesli (no sugar) Whole wheat bread crumbs **Freezer:** Strawberries Blueberries Raspberries Shrimp Organic mixed vegetables Sweet corn **Refrigerator:** Miso paste

PHASE TWO: Muscle Building & Fitness

Weekly Menu & Shopping List

Week 2:

Meal	Day 1	Day 2	Day 3	Day 4	Day 5	Day 6	Day 7
Breakfast	Oatmeal & egg white pancakes Juiceplus Fruit Fish Oil	Toasted oatmeal w/apple, almond & banana Juiceplus Fruit Fish Oil	Blueberry-mango smoothie Juiceplus Fruit Fish Oil	Spinach-tomato egg white scramble Juiceplus Fruit Fish Oil	Cottage cheese & yogurt with blueberries Juiceplus Fruit Fish Oil	Yogurt parfait Juiceplus Fruit Fish Oil	Free Day
Lunch	Salmon wrap w/ orange chili sauce Juiceplus Vineyard	Chicken, blueberry walnut rice salad Juiceplus Vineyard	Seared ahi tuna salad w/wasabi vinaigrette Juiceplus Vineyard	Thai style chicken rice wrap Juiceplus Vineyard	California chicken salad Juiceplus Vineyard	Escarole & white bean soup Juiceplus Vineyard	
Afternoon	Hard-boiled egg whites & sliced apples	Orange & 16 almonds	Cottage cheese, yogurt & blueberries	1 piece fruit 1 tsp almond butter	Peanutty hummus & sliced apple	Smoked salmon w/ edamame	
Dinner	Chicken in red wine sauce Juiceplus Veggie Fish oil	Steak & asparagus stir-fry Juiceplus Veggie Fish oil	Cod w/chili, garlic, ginger sauce Juiceplus Veggie Fish oil	Black pepper chicken Juiceplus Veggie Fish oil	Ground beef & cabbage Juiceplus Veggie Fish oil	Lime-ginger pan-seared sole Juiceplus Veggie Fish oil	

Week Two Shopping List & Other Necessities:

Shopping List	Precooked	Pantry necessities
Chicken breast Salmon fillet Ahi tuna smoked salmon Cod Eggs Ground turkey Lean ground beef Canned chickpeas Cottage cheese Greek plain non-fat yogurt Steak Soft silken tofu Firm tofu Low fat cottage cheese Mild salsa Rice paper wrappers (Asian market) Tahini **Fruits:** Apples Oranges Bananas Strawberries Grapefruit Grapefruit Broccoli **Vegetables:** Spinach Tomatoes Avocado Red bell pepper Garlic Onions Green onions Large head of lettuce Mushrooms Cilantro Ginger Broccoli Cabbage Asparagus Lemon & lime Bean sprouts Baby greens Romaine lettuce Cucumber Carrots	Brown rice Chicken breast Turkey breast	Black-eyed peas Canned tuna Canned salmon Canned black beans Canned kidney beans Canned white beans Canned pinto beans Old fashioned oats Soymilk (unsweetened) Raisins Meal Replacement: JuicePlus Complete Ground flax meal Peanut/almond butter Sliced almonds Walnuts Canned diced tomatoes Tomato paste Whole wheat flour Natural muesli (no sugar) Whole wheat bread crumbs **Freezer:** Strawberries Blueberries Raspberries Shrimp Scallops Organic mixed vegetables Sweet corn **Refrigerator:** Miso paste

Week 3:

Meal	Day 1	Day 2	Day 3	Day 4	Day 5	Day 6	Day 7
Breakfast	Chicken hash Juiceplus Fruit Fish Oil	Chocolate peanut butter oatmeal Juiceplus Fruit Fish Oil	Egg white scramble w/ spinach & tomatoes Juiceplus Fruit Fish Oil	Strawber-rilicious smoothie Juiceplus Fruit Fish Oil	Yogurt parfait Juiceplus Fruit Fish Oil	Oatmeal & egg whites pancakes Juiceplus Fruit Fish Oil	Free Day
Lunch	Turkey stir-fry Juiceplus Vineyard	Chicken patties w/ chili sauce Juiceplus Vineyard	Curry chicken salad Juiceplus Vineyard	Chicken fajita lettuce wrap Juiceplus Vineyard	Three bean salad Juiceplus Vineyard	Chicken & lentils w/ spinach & tomatoes Juiceplus Vineyard	
Afternoon	Peanutty hummus & sliced apple	Apple & 16 almonds	Yogurt & berries	1 piece fruit 1 tsp almond butter	Hard-boiled egg whites & orange	Quick home-made chicken soup	
Dinner	Stir-fry black pepper beef Juiceplus Veggie Fish oil	Citrus salmon w/ white beans Juiceplus Veggie Fish oil	Asian beef stir-fry Juiceplus Veggie Fish oil	Shrimp & scallops w/ spinach Juiceplus Veggie Fish oil	Halibut w/ tomato-wine sauce Juiceplus Veggie Fish oil	Brazillian black bean stew Juiceplus Veggie Fish oil	

Week Three Shopping List & Other Necessities:

Shopping List	Precooked	Pantry necessities
Chicken breast Salmon fillet Halibut Frozen shrimp Eggs Ground turkey Cottage cheese Greek plain nonfat yogurt Scallops Steak Soft silken tofu Firm tofu Low fat cottage cheese Mild salsa Rice paper wrappers (Asian market) Tahini **Fruits:** Apples Oranges Bananas Strawberries **Vegetables:** Spinach Tomatoes Avocado Red bell pepper Garlic Onions Green onions Large head of lettuce Mushrooms Cilantro Ginger Grapefruit Broccoli Potato Peach Ripe mango Sweet potato Shiitake mushroom	Brown rice Chicken breast Turkey breast	Black-eyed peas Canned tuna Canned salmon Canned black beans Canned kidney beans Canned white beans Canned pinto beans Canned lentils Old fashioned oats Soymilk (unsweetened) Raisins Protein Powder (JuicePlus Complete) Ground flax meal Peanut/almond butter Sliced almonds Canned diced tomatoes Tomato paste Whole wheat flour Natural muesli (no sugar) Whole wheat bread crumbs Sesame seeds **Freezer:** Strawberries Blueberries Raspberries Shrimp Organic mixed vegetables Sweet corn Mango **Refrigerator:** Miso paste Pickled ginger

PHASE THREE: Fat Loss (2 Weeks)

During the Fat Loss Phase of your program you want to reduce your daily caloric intake by 15%-20%. Even though the research suggests that any macronutrient ratio (protein, carbs, fat) is just as effective in facilitating fat loss, 20 years of experience has taught me differently.

I have found that reducing your carbohydrate intake such that dietary fat becomes your primary energy source to be the most effective. The research does also suggest that a diet of 22% fat increased the use of stored body fat by about 20%, in comparison to a low-fat, high carbohydrate diet (American Journal of Physiology, Endocrinology & Metabolism).

Therefore, on this phase of your program, I recommend cutting back (not eliminating them) on the carbohydrates and eating more protein and healthy fats.

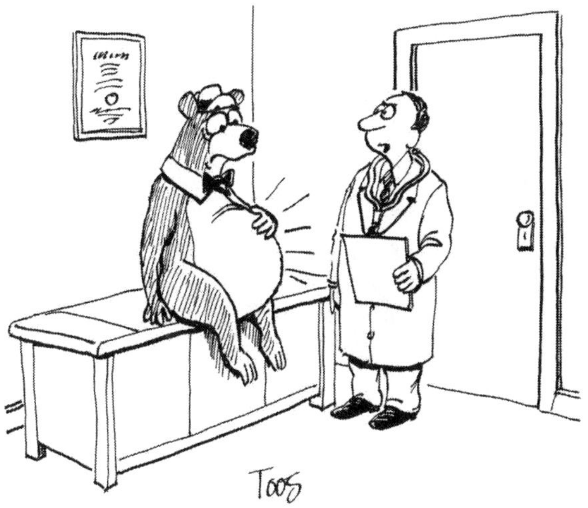

"You gotta cut back on the pic-a-nic baskets."

Phase Three: Fat Loss Daily Meal Plan:

1200 Calories

Meal	Carbohydrate	Protein	Fat	Vegetable	Fruit
Breakfast	1	1	1		1
Lunch		1	1	2	
Afternoon		1	1		2
Dinner		1	1	2	

EXAMPLE:

Breakfast	Lunch	Mid-Afternoon	Dinner
1/2 cup oatmeal 2 egg whites 1 whole egg 1/2 cup blueberries 1 tsp peanut butter Supplement: 2 Juiceplus fruit capsules; fish oil	4 oz chicken breast 1 cup broccoli Supplement: 2 Juiceplus vine-yard capsules; fish oil	1 cup berries 12-15 almonds	4 oz fish 1 cup asparagus 1/2 small avocado Supplement: 2 Juiceplus vegetable cap-sules; fish oil

1500 Calories

Meal	Carbohydrate	Protein	Fat	Vegetable	Fruit
Breakfast	1	1	1		1
Lunch		2	1	2	
Afternoon		1	1		2
Dinner		1	1	2	

EXAMPLE:

Breakfast	Lunch	Mid-Afternoon	Dinner
1/2 cup oatmeal 2 egg whites 1 whole egg 1/2 cup blueberries 1 tsp peanut butter Supplement: 2 Juiceplus fruit capsules; fish oil	8 oz chicken breast 1 cup broccoli Supplement: 2 Juiceplus vine-yard capsules; fish oil	4 oz turkey breast 1 sliced apple 1 tsp peanut butter	4 oz fish 1 cup asparagus 1/2 small avocado Supplement: 2 Juiceplus vegetable cap-sules; fish oil

1800 Calories

Meal	Carbohydrate	Protein	Fat	Vegetable	Fruit
Breakfast	1	1	1		1
Lunch		2	1	2	
Afternoon		2	1		2
Dinner		2	1	2	
Anytime		2	1		1

EXAMPLE:

Breakfast	Lunch	Mid-Afternoon	Dinner	Anytime
1/2 cup oatmeal 2 egg whites 1 whole egg 1/2 cup blueberries 1 tsp peanut butter Supplement: 2 Juiceplus fruit capsules; fish oil	8 oz chicken breast 1 cup broccoli Supplement: 2 Juiceplus vineyard capsules; fish oil	4 oz turkey breast 1 sliced apple 1 tsp peanut butter	6 oz fish 1 cup asparagus 1/2 small avocado Supplement: 2 Juiceplus vegetable capsules; fish oil	3 hardboiled egg whites 1 tsp peanut butter 1 orange

2000 Calories

Meal	Carbohydrate	Protein	Fat	Vegetable	Fruit
Breakfast	1	2	1		1
Lunch		2	2	2	
Afternoon		2	1		2
Dinner		2	2	2	
Anytime		2	1		2

EXAMPLE:

Breakfast	Lunch	Mid-Afternoon	Dinner	Anytime
1/2 cup oatmeal 4 egg whites 2 whole eggs 1/2 cup blueberries Supplement: 2 Juiceplus fruit capsules; fish oil	8 oz chicken breast 1 cup broccoli Supplement: 2 Juiceplus vineyard capsules; fish oil	4 oz turkey breast 1 sliced apple 1 tsp peanut butter	6 oz fish 1 cup asparagus 1/2 small avocado Supplement: 2 Juiceplus vegetable capsules; fish oil	4 hardboiled egg whites 1 tsp peanut butter 1 orange 1 small banana

PHASE 3: Fat Loss

2-WEEK MEAL PLAN

Note: All the recipes for the meal plan are in **Dr. Del's Rapid Fatloss Cookbook.**

Week 1:

Meal	Day 1	Day 2	Day 3	Day 4	Day 5	Day 6	Day 7
Breakfast	Toasted Oatmeal w/apple, almonds & banana Juiceplus Fruit Fish Oil	Chicken hash Juiceplus Fruit Fish Oil	Blueberry-mango smoothie Juiceplus Fruit Fish Oil	Spinach-tomato egg white scramble Juiceplus Fruit Fish Oil	Chocolate peanut butter oatmeal Juiceplus Fruit Fish Oil	Breakfast bowl Juiceplus Fruit Fish Oil	Choose any fatloss meal
Lunch	Salmon wrap w/ orange chili sauce Juiceplus Vineyard	Spiced beef & onions wrap Juiceplus Vineyard	Seared ahi tuna salad w/wasabi vinaigrette Juiceplus Vineyard	Thai style chicken rice paper wrap Juiceplus Vineyard	California chicken salad Juiceplus Vineyard	Sesame chicken tenders & arugula salad Juiceplus Vineyard	
Afternoon	Sliced apple & 16 almonds/ cashews	Orange & 16 almonds	Sliced apple &16 almonds/ cashews	1 piece fruit & 1 tsp almond butter	Peanutty hummus & sliced apple	Sliced apple &16 almonds/ cashews	
Dinner	Chicken in red wine sauce Juiceplus Veggie Fish oil	Steak & asparagus stir-fry Juiceplus Veggie Fish oil	Cod w/chili, garlic, ginger sauce Juiceplus Veggie Fish oil	Black pepper chicken Juiceplus Veggie Fish oil	Ground beef & cabbage Juiceplus Veggie Fish oil	Lime-ginger pan-seared sole Juiceplus Veggie Fish oil	

FATLOSS MEAL PLAN

Week 2:

Meal	Day 1	Day 2	Day 3	Day 4	Day 5	Day 6	Day 7
Breakfast	Toasted Oatmeal w/apple, almonds & banana Juiceplus Fruit Fish Oil	Chicken hash Juiceplus Fruit Fish Oil	Blueberry-mango smoothie Juiceplus Fruit Fish Oil	Spinach-tomato egg white scramble Juiceplus Fruit Fish Oil	Chocolate peanut butter oatmeal Juiceplus Fruit Fish Oil	Breakfast bowl Juiceplus Fruit Fish Oil	Choose any fatloss meal
Lunch	Salmon wrap w/ orange chili sauce Juiceplus Vineyard	Spiced beef & onions wrap Juiceplus Vineyard	Seared ahi tuna salad w/wasabi vinaigrette Juiceplus Vineyard	Thai style chicken rice paper wrap Juiceplus Vineyard	California chicken salad Juiceplus Vineyard	Sesame chicken tenders & arugula salad Juiceplus Vineyard	
Afternoon	Sliced apple & 16 almonds/ cashews	Orange & 16 almonds	Sliced apple &16 almonds/ cashews	1 piece fruit & 1 tsp almond butter	Peanutty hummus & sliced apple	Sliced apple &16 almonds/ cashews	
Dinner	Baked tilapia w/ orange tomato sauce Juiceplus Veggie Fish oil	Steak & asparagus stir-fry Juiceplus Veggie Fish oil	Cod w/chili, garlic, ginger sauce Juiceplus Veggie Fish oil	Black pepper chicken Juiceplus Veggie Fish oil	Orange zest salmon Juiceplus Veggie Fish oil	Lime-ginger pan-seared sole Juiceplus Veggie Fish oil	

The Key to Your Success:

Strive for Consistency, Not Perfection!

Perfection doesn't exist; it's a fairytale. Therefore, don't beat yourself up when you slip up. Don't lose any sleep over it, just recommit yourself to your program and move on. The truth is it happens to the best of us. It's called life happens.

We all fall off the wagon from time to time, the secret is to get up and get right back on. If you miss a meal or eat something that's not a part of your plan, forget about it. Recommit to your plan at your next meal.

If you miss a few days of working out, recommit as quickly as you can and strive to be consistent.

Of course, if you find that you're consistently being inconsistent with your plan, you need to have a serious look at why things are not working. What's going on in your life that is pulling you away from your commitment to yourself?

As I've said many times, if you try to fit a program into your already chaotic life, there's a greater chance that you will fail. You need to reorganize your life around your goals. This is assuming that health and fitness is one of your top values. If it isn't, you will struggle.

Don't get discouraged when you have a bad week. Put it behind you and come up with a better plan for the week starting today.

Most people that I speak with struggle with their meal plan because they never take the time to prepare. Everything begins with preparation. Would you give an important business presentation to top executives at your company without first preparing for it? I don't think so.

There are 168 hours in a week. If you sleep 7 hours each night, that leaves 119 hours. Even if you work ten hours each day, seven days per week, there are still 49 hours unaccounted for. You only need about two to three hours each week to shop and prepare your meals for the entire week.

So what's your excuse?

If you can't make time to go shopping, find a few places in your area with menu items that will allow you to stay on your meal plan.

If that doesn't work, then just continue to allow your life to be the boss of you. You're not ready for what it takes to get results. That doesn't mean that you should give up; don't do that. However, you need to change your expectations of what's possible.

You don't have to be perfect to get great results. But you do need to have a plan and you must follow that plan more than you deviate from it.

The more you deviate from your plan, the longer it will take you to get the results you're looking for. The more you stick to your plan, the faster you will reach your goal.

Success is nothing more than doing small things consistently over time. You don't have to be perfect, however, you do have to be consistent.

You can do it, so go for it!

"Success is consistency over time."

About the Author

Del Millers, PhD
Author, Speaker, Life Coach

DEL THE AUTHOR

Other Books by Del Millers:

DR. DEL'S RAPID FATLOSS MANUAL:
A Scientific Approach to Building Your Leanest Body Ever

DR. DEL'S RAPID FATLOSS COOKBOOK:
Quick & Easy "10-Minute Meals" for Building Your Leanest Body Ever.

DR. DEL'S RAPID FATLOSS DETOX-CLEANSE PROGRAM:
A 21-Day Whole Food Based Plan for
Jumpstarting Your Body's Fat-Burning System.

SIMPLY DELICIOUS:
Quick & Easy 10-Minute "Fit" Recipes
and Nutrition Guide.

DEL'S 10-MINUTE TOTAL BODY WORKOUT:
When all you've got is 10 minutes to spare!

DANCING WITH GOD:
How you can Make Exercise
a Playful Adventure of Body and Soul!

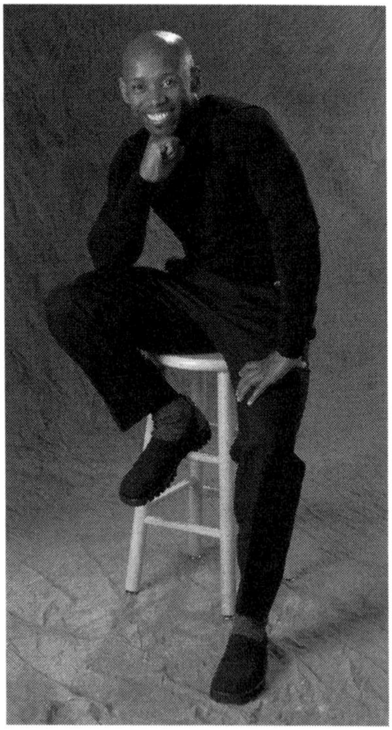

DEL THE SPEAKER

Speaking Engagements And Seminars:

Speaking the Spirit of the Body's Wisdom

When Del Millers speaks, people listen. He knows an awful lot about the physical body, and he looks like it. He also knows an awful lot about the mind and emotions, and he demonstrates it. And that he has a very intimate and personal relationship with his own spiritual nature puts him in a very unique position to be able to support, motivate, and encourage people to reach new levels with their personal dreams and ambitions. As one client puts it, "I have had many personal fitness trainers and many dance and tennis teachers. Del is the first one to really help me reach my goals. He's tough and demanding and kind at the same time. He knows what he's doing; he's an expert."

Del has been extremely successful as a motivational speaker and coach because he addresses all aspects of the human being. He is intelligent, well spoken, and engaging, whether he's exploring the many aspects of health and nutrition or describing how exercise is really like dancing with God. He fascinates audiences and individuals alike because he practices what he preaches. He is a happy man with a firm grasp on his reality—and he assists others to reach the same amazing place. He is, in a word, inspiring.

Del holds a Masters Degree in Spiritual Psychology, a degree he earned by demonstrating self-mastery, and a Ph.D. in Nutritional Sciences. He is also an accomplished writer, poet, and performer as well as a master instructor of Kung Fu and Tai Chi Chuan, a Personal Fitness Coach and a sought after corporate consultant. Del is truly a pioneer, combining the fields of Fitness and Transformation.

Del Millers is a powerhouse, standing on a solid foundation of education and experience. When he speaks, people want what he's got. The good news is, he knows how to deliver.

PRIVATE CONSULTATION

Dr. Del is available for phone or email fitness, nutrition and life coaching.

Del's Contact Information:

For consultations or to book Del for a seminar or speaking engagement, please contact:

DEL MILLERS

Del Millers International
10736 Jefferson Blvd. #693
Culver City, CA 90230
USA

http://www.delmillers.com
del@delmillers.com
1-888-800-9463

Subscribe to Dr. Del's FREE Email Newsletter:
www.drdelmillers.com

Subscribe to Dr. Del's Blog:
www.drdelblog.com

Dr. Del's Online Fitness & Nutrition Coaching Program:
Get a FREE Fitness Analysis and One-Month Membership
www.personalfitness.com

Join the conversation online:

FACEBOOK **Facebook.com/drdelmillers**
Like Dr Del for daily updates and postings

TWITTER **@drdelmillers**
Stay connected

YouTube **Youtube.com/drdelmillers**
Visit Dr. Del's video channel

DEL MILLERS INTERNATIONAL

Inspiration, Support & Encouragement,
For Your Personal Growth and Transformation!
http://www.delmillers.com

"Whether you think you can
or you think you can't, you're right."

~ *Henry Ford*

"I don't have a message,
my life is my message."

~ Mahatma Gandhi

Made in United States
Troutdale, OR
07/25/2026

51590719R00035